Healing Mental Illness
A Pilgrimage From Birth To Home

For Dad and Mom

Preface

Everyone has something to offer the community. The puzzle of life, as I see it, is to figure out what it is that a person has to offer.

This book documents my process of figuring out what I have to offer. My pilgrimage has been both exhausting and humbling. Since 1980 I have been focusing on myself. I am not apologizing for that reality. I have been on red alert and in crisis mode in a struggle to survive for the past thirty-three years. I appreciate the validation for this effort that I received from Nicky: "Danny, this is big. This kind of research SAVES LIVES!"

I am selling to you the insights that I have accumulated over time so that you can use them, possibly, to enhance your own pilgrimage. What I have received for free is available to you, too, for free. What I am asking you to pay money for is my story, my wisdom and the details of my application of what I have learned to the problems that I have had during my life.

I am not able to heal you. I am not a doctor and the things that I have done along my journey are specific to me. I took risks with my own life in exercising my own personal liberty.

My suggestion is that anyone who desires to be healed of mental illness should cooperate closely with professionals who have been trained and authorized to treat the mind, the body and the spirit. That's what I did. The positive results that I have enjoyed have come to me as a blessing beyond my doing.

So, what do you have to offer?

Introduction

In 1980, at the age of fourteen, I told my parents I believed that there was something wrong with me. As I remember, the conversation took place in the kitchen of our house. During the thirty-three years between then and now, both of my parents sacrificially invested themselves in my well-being. The pilgrimage I have walked so far has been an experience of the love that a parent has for a child.

Today I am able to testify to a healing from mental illness.

By "healing" I mean an improvement in my well-being. I measure this improvement by observing myself and reflecting on how well, or how not-so-well, I manage the daily demands of my life. Social services have questionnaires that, over time, show improvements, or declines, in functional areas and subjective emotional states.

By being public with my story I am cementing the improvements through accountability. Backsliding will make me look foolish so by going on record about the before-and-after of both my interior and exterior lives I will put pressure on myself to live in the healing.

Also, I have not appreciated the gift of life and the cards I have been dealt as much as I should have given the circumstances that I have survived. Ironically, the same problem that hindered my success has clouded my perspective to see just how successful my life has really been so far.

What is it that makes parents sacrifice themselves for the benefit of their children?

Chapter One: Problem?

Something is wrong. Why am I alone? My awareness of my adolescent self in 1980 was that I did not connect with what was going on around me. There was something wrong with the way that I interacted with people. I grew up in a large family. I knew that I was loved.

Everyone has problems that are important to them, individually. Birth, at best, can be difficult for anyone. Pilgrims enter a new land where others are already living. When I arrived, my parents already had seventeen years of experience with their family life.

At the age of two I experienced a medical trauma. An electrolyte loss in my body caused me to become very sick. I experienced a seizure, of a few hours' duration. The records report that I regained consciousness six hours after intravenous treatment was begun. When I had arrived at the hospital I was semi-comatose, with muscular weakness on the right side of my body, attributable to compromised brain function.

Family mythology attributes this to "heart sickness" due to emotional sensitivity. I make quick, strong bonds with people. Later in life I would learn the difficulties that this would cause for me in relationships. I am very fortunate to possess medical records from this time in my life. As an adult I have benefitted from knowing about the objective details of this crisis and the possible after-effects upon my cognition. The implications must have been unimaginable at the time.

During my adolescence I spent a lot of time alone. I avoided eye contact.

I grew up in a big house with lots of space. Most of my life I had my own bedroom. I enjoyed being alone in my quiet room. Often I would rearrange my room furniture. It was like a new beginning.

Chapter Two: Solution?

I'm curious. Can this problem be solved? Is healing possible? My father was a maintenance man. He fixed things. If he couldn't fix something then he just put gray tape on it. The sacrifices that my father made so that his family was cared for are numerous. The work that I have done during the past thirty-three years of healing has been difficult at times. Having grown up around a Dad who worked, I know what work is and I am not unwilling to work.

I believe that every problem has a solution. I am curious about people. At UMass the only textbook that I read cover-to-cover was the Human Resources course textbook. If my brain had been damaged by the seizure I had to find out how I could compensate for it.

At the age of six I experienced another medical trauma. A sore throat and fever failed to subside when I received treatment at a local hospital. I developed severe respiratory distress. By the time the thoracic surgeon got to me in the Operating Room I was in extremus, cyanotic and flaccid. Not a good situation for a six year old boy who had been semi-comatose during a six hour seizure just four years earlier! What happened next?!

As I write this the goose bumps are discharging the stress from deep within my body. I believe that you, too, can let go of your trauma and receive a healing. That is why I am selling these insights to you. I cannot heal you but maybe my story will inspire you to keep looking for your truth and solution.

So, what happened next? The surgeon performed an emergency bedside tracheotomy and I was transferred to a larger hospital. The ambulance sped through traffic, over the bridge and into the city. Upon arrival I was severely hypoxic and agitated. Air. I need air! Now!

For as long as I can remember I have been protective of my neck and my access to air. Even when I smoked cigarettes. Crazy, huh? This is a book about healing mental illness, remember?

Manual ventilation in the emergency room left me with bilateral pneumothoraxes and significant pneumomediastinum. The tracheotomy tube had come out of place, maybe during the frantic ambulance ride through difficult traffic, and the positive ventilation had filled my chest up with air instead of my lungs.

So, I survived round two, by the grace of God. The records state that no formal neurological testing was done at the time. I was in first grade. When I reached third grade in school I would visit the Resource Room (Special Education, at the time). In my thirties a vocational counselor would evaluate me and suggest that my intellectual performance indicated "slow psychomotor speed."

I have been spared from any negative feelings towards anyone involved in my childhood traumas. Here I am now. Trying to help you by encouraging you to learn your own story and find a solution to the problem that is keeping you unsatisfied.

Is there something that you are still angry about?

Chapter Three: Desire

I want a better life. My desires have driven my behaviors for as long as I can remember. Sometimes the behavior was bad. Most of the time my behavior matched my good intentions. In 1980 when I alerted my parents to my sense of having a problem, I intended that they should fix it like the "fixed" everything else in my life.

What do you want? I want to be healed.

In my twenties, the first vocational counselor to examine me found a large number of solid thinking abilities including vocabulary and reading comprehension within the superior range of the scales used for the testing. He also noted that there was continued, long term anxiety that effected how well I perform. I went to a vocational counselor because an acquaintance had heard me speak at a support group meeting and suggested that I had ADD because my story was all over the place and hard to follow. She told me that vocational counseling had helped her. She had a job. This is about twenty-five years after the second childhood trauma during which I nearly suffocated on the operating table. Another eight years later a third vocational counselor would conclude that I may have high-functioning Asperger's syndrome.

People who have helped you along the way?

_____

_____

_____

The first vocational assessment in my twenties started to link my cognition to my mental health and failure to make anything of myself with my Bachelor's degree from college education.

I began attending a support group because of the pain. My refrain was "My life hurts." I wasn't getting what I wanted. Things were slipping further out of reach. I lost things that I had started with or had accumulated along the way.

Has this happened to you?

Chapter Four: Read To Me

I like to read. I like to learn. People tell me that I am a good teacher. My identity is strongest when I am sharing knowledge with people and transmitting to them the power to take action to improve their lives like I was blessed to have done myself.

Reading is freedom, I think. Reading at my own pace and processing at my own speed is comfortable.   Blasts of knowledge for a confused mind have helped me to make connections and synthesize data relevant to my struggle. Having questions answered is a form of healing. Knowledge supports mental health, I think.

As a child learning to read I would read to my father at bedtime. I have a great picture that my sister took of me reading to my Dad in my bed. He's asleep. I hope to include that picture in the next edition of this book.

Over the years, the ability to read well has been critical to my pilgrimage. Libraries have attracted me because they are quiet. Being in a place with so many answers was often positively therapeutic for me as I struggled to understand what was happening to me. I went down many blind alleys, sometimes arriving at dead ends, but the research training was beneficial. Now I understand the concepts of primary and secondary sources. I am comfortable developing and expressing my own point of view as seen through my own life's lens.

Listening to books on tape has also been a beneficial experience. It seems that I learn better when it occurs in conjunction with some physical activity. Audio books enabled me to learn quickly and deeply.

Chapter Five: Equality

It's not fair. I was the youngest with a sixteen year spread between me and the oldest. During adolescence I watched and participated in lives that were beyond my "now" at the time: high school, college, working, marriage and child-rearing. I often became inappropriately absorbed into those identities because of poor personal boundaries on my part. At the time I had no idea what role the brain plays in determining where I stop and you begin.

Are all people really created equal? My motivation for trying to receive healing was that I wanted the life that I saw other people having all around me. Because I perceived and believed that there was something wrong with me I handicapped myself. Everyone has different abilities. How I processed my failures dramatically influenced the development of my self esteem. I had no idea, as I do now, that my cognitive processing was somehow faulty due to brain damage possibly caused by childhood trauma. It all seemed so normal to me.

As I aged into adult life it became apparent to me that I was not tracking (keeping up and succeeding). A series of jobs without a career path indicated to me that there was a problem. Maybe I wasn't equal after all? I continued to pursue each insight and also to maintain any progress that I could make.

At the beginning of this book, in the Preface, I said, "Everyone has something to offer." I was puzzled by my inability to imitate the success of others. I did not understand that they were succeeding at the application of their unique gifts. I needed to find my own calling.

Chapter Six: Help!

I enjoy helping other people. As an adolescent and young adult I often felt lonely. I felt disconnected from my peers. Social interaction with family and friends did not have the depth and intimacy that I thought in my mind that it should have had.

I myself need help. I am sometimes too empathetic. My brain functions in such a way that when I interact with people I could imagine being them with a little too much detail for my own good. Poor personal boundaries on my part have caused me a lot of wasted time and lost resources, even if I did help that other person with their own problems. It's a mystery to me how the lines get drawn.

Mental illness is defined by diagnostic criteria. Healing the mental illness of Borderline Personality Disorder (BPD) is a rare occurrence. At this point in time on my pilgrimage the healing surged dramatically forward and upward.

The BPD criteria played out in my life like this: my identity was fluid, my sense of self varied and I had a difficult time maintaining appropriate boundaries between myself and others. I would come to learn, over time, that I actually appropriated aspects of personalities external to myself in order to fill in the gaps in who I thought I was. Weird, huh? I still don't understand it so don't be discouraged if it makes no sense to you either.

This book, in each succeeding edition, is about healing mental illness. The issue of identity is at the root of the tree, I think, of my mental illness. My interior life is continually influenced by my experiences with the outside world. Faulty cognition and hyper-sensitive neurology made my relationship with the outside world exhausting. I saw myself as unable to cope.

Chapter Seven: Resting Meditation

At various times along this pilgrimage I have had a variety of living situations and work schedules that have provided varying degrees of opportunity for rest. At my worst, when I would get overwhelmed, there would inevitably be some physical health crisis. I would decide to prioritize my recovery from the current ailment as best I knew how. I would quit whatever job I had at the time.

There was one particular time, not long after my nearly-not graduation from college, a particular time when I reasoned that it did not make sense to suffer through work life now and enjoy retirement later. I wanted to be out of physical misery now even if it meant poverty and/or underemployment. My desire to be pain-free was paramount in my thinking. This reasoning was okay in my twenties when I had resources to fall back on in a pinch.

As I got deeper into my thirties, however, it became clear to me that I must work, no matter what the physical consequences would be, so that I could achieve independence from my parents.

I did not comprehend at the time that there was a direct connection between my physical problems, my mental health problems and my neurology that had been, possibly, damaged at ages two and six.

Like many people, I guess, spirituality sustained me through many dark days. My mind was full of religious chaos that hindered my progress. As I focused on taking responsibility for my body, my mind and my spirit, there were several moments of severe crisis. The existential angst was, at times, overwhelming. In future editions I will tell some amazing stories about some of the things that have happened to me over the past thirty-three years. Stay tuned.

One particular situation involved the issue of psychiatric medication. I take medication and I recommend that persons to whom a medical professional suggests medication, I recommend that the person take the medication, as prescribed, like I did, and cooperate with the help being offered.

But there was a time when a person challenged my "reliance" on meds and I had to leave a social community. Later, I became able to stop taking the medication, under medical supervision, and I have not taken that medication again.

I tell this story because in this situation I had to be strong and very courageous and trust, through faith, that staying on the meds was the right thing to do at the time. I was sad to leave that social community but my life is so good now that I rarely even remember that person now. I wish them well. Peace.

A Final Word About Friendship

I believe that people need healthy relationships. We need family, friends, peers and community. For most of my life, so far, I have had a lack of skill in interacting with others. I have tended to dominate conversations with running dialogue about my area of interest. Frequently I have repeated sentences. Frequently I have repeated sentences. See what I mean?

The next edition of this book will include more information about how friendships make life worth living...from birth to home.

I don't think that it is good to be alone. I have not enjoyed being alone during those times when I really wanted someone to be with me and share in what was happening in my life at that time.

Do you feel alone?

Conclusion

and

Preface to the Second Edition

There is a fundamental legal phrase known as "time is of the essence." This phrase means that if something is not done at, or within, a specified time, there could be irreversible damage to someone.

Do you remember in Chapter Two when you read the words, "Air. I need air! Now!" during the description of my childhood crisis? Well, my hunch is that if this book has gotten into your hands then there may be something that you need to do. And now is the time.

I am emphasizing the drama of the pilgrimage because the outcome could be dramatic, too, if you act now. But what if you have multiple things pending and do not know what to do first? In the second edition we will talk more about setting priorities. See you then! Dan

The End (of edition one)

www.ingramcontent.com/pod-product-compliance
Lightning Source LLC
Chambersburg PA
CBHW060708280326
41933CB00012B/2344